Wall Pilates Awesome Guide for Beginners

Advancing Your Wall Pilates Practice

By

Keaton Macallister

Copyright@2023

Table of Contents

CHAPTER 1

Introduction

1.1 What is Pilates?

Pilates is a holistic and systematic approach to physical fitness and well-being that was developed by Joseph H. Pilates in the early 20th century. Born out of a fusion of influences, including yoga, martial arts, and gymnastics, Pilates is designed to enhance physical strength, flexibility, balance, and mental awareness. Its fundamental principles emphasize core strength, controlled movements, precision, concentration, and proper breathing techniques.

At its core, Pilates is not just a series of exercises; it's a philosophy of movement that encourages the development of a strong mind-body connection. Joseph Pilates himself once described his method as "the complete coordination of body, mind, and spirit." The focus on the mind-body connection is one of the distinguishing features that sets Pilates apart from other forms of exercise.

Pilates exercises are typically performed in a controlled and flowing manner, with an emphasis on the quality of each movement rather than the quantity. The method can be adapted to accommodate people of all ages and fitness levels, making it a versatile practice that can be tailored to individual needs.

In traditional Pilates, exercises are usually done on a mat or with the use of various specialized equipment, such as the Reformer, Cadillac, and Wunda Chair. However, in recent years, the concept of Wall Pilates has gained attention as an innovative and effective approach to the practice. Wall Pilates introduces a unique element to the traditional method by utilizing a wall for support, resistance, and alignment in various exercises.

1.2 Benefits of Wall Pilates

Wall Pilates, like its traditional counterpart, offers a multitude of benefits that extend to physical, mental, and even emotional well-being. These advantages make it an appealing and accessible option for individuals of all fitness levels, especially beginners.

Here are some of the key benefits of Wall Pilates:

1. Enhanced Core Strength: Wall Pilates places a strong emphasis on engaging the core muscles. The wall provides stability and support, allowing beginners to focus on building core strength without feeling overwhelmed. Over time, this increased core strength can lead to better posture, reduced lower back pain, and improved overall stability.

2. Improved Alignment: The wall serves as a reliable reference point for proper alignment during exercises. This is particularly beneficial for beginners who may struggle with maintaining correct alignment when performing Pilates movements. By using the wall as a guide, individuals can enhance their body awareness and alignment.

3. Increased Flexibility: Wall Pilates incorporates stretches and movements that can contribute to increased flexibility over time. These stretches, when performed with the wall's support, help improve joint mobility and reduce the risk of injury.

4. Stress Reduction: The focus on controlled breathing and mindfulness in Wall Pilates provides a calming and stress-reducing effect. Practitioners often find that Wall Pilates can be a meditative practice, offering an escape from the demands and pressures of daily life.

5. Accessible to Beginners: Wall Pilates is particularly accessible to beginners because of the support and guidance offered by the wall. It provides a gradual introduction to Pilates, allowing individuals to become familiar with the exercises and principles at their own pace.

6. Versatility: Wall Pilates can be adapted to various fitness levels and goals. Whether you are looking for a gentle introduction to exercise, a way to rehabilitate from an injury, or a challenging workout, Wall Pilates can be customized to meet your needs.

7. Enhanced Body Awareness: Wall Pilates encourages a heightened sense of body awareness. Practitioners become attuned to their movements, posture, and breathing, which can translate into improved overall physical awareness and coordination in daily life.

Wall Pilates is a variant of the traditional Pilates method that offers numerous advantages, making it an ideal choice for beginners and anyone looking to enhance their physical fitness and well-being. The wall's support and guidance facilitate a gentle entry into the world of Pilates, while still delivering the core principles and benefits that make Pilates a respected and enduring fitness practice. This guide will explore these benefits in greater detail and provide a roadmap for incorporating Wall Pilates into your life.

CHAPTER 2

Getting Started

2.1 Setting up Your Space

Before diving into Wall Pilates, it's essential to prepare a suitable space for your practice. A well-organized and inviting environment can enhance your experience and ensure safety. Here's how to set up your space for Wall Pilates:

Clear the Area: Begin by clearing the space where you intend to practice

Wall Pilates. Remove any obstacles or clutter that might interfere with your movements. A clean and unobstructed area will reduce the risk of accidents and help you focus on your exercises.

Wall Selection: Choose a wall that is clean and free from any protruding objects. The wall should be sturdy and capable of supporting your body weight during exercises. Ensure that it is in good condition and free from any structural issues.

Lighting: Adequate lighting is crucial for safety and concentration. Ensure that your practice space is well-lit. Natural light is ideal, but if that's not possible, consider using bright, warm lighting to create a welcoming atmosphere.

Ventilation: Proper ventilation is important to keep your practice space comfortable. Good airflow can help you stay cool and prevent overheating during your workouts. If your space is indoors, ensure it is well-ventilated.

Music and Ambiance: Many people find that playing soothing music or creating a calming atmosphere enhances their Pilates practice. Consider adding some background music or using essential oils or incense to create a pleasant ambiance.

2.2 Necessary Equipment

Wall Pilates is known for its simplicity, but there are a few pieces of equipment and props that can be beneficial, especially for beginners. Here are some items you might want to consider having on hand:

Yoga Mat: While Wall Pilates doesn't require a mat like traditional Pilates, having a yoga mat can provide comfort and support when doing floor exercises and stretches.

Resistance Bands: Resistance bands can be used to add intensity to certain exercises and provide additional support for your movements. They are particularly helpful for beginners looking to build strength gradually.

Pilates Ball: A small inflatable Pilates ball can be used for various exercises, including core work and balance training. It's an excellent addition to your Wall Pilates toolkit.

Water Bottle: Staying hydrated during your practice is important. Have a water bottle nearby to sip on between exercises.

Comfortable Attire: Wear comfortable, breathable clothing that allows for a full range of motion. Avoid clothes with zippers, buttons, or other elements that might dig into your skin or restrict movement.

Footwear: In Wall Pilates, you typically practice barefoot or in grip socks, which provide traction on the floor. Regular shoes are not required and are often discouraged to maintain a better connection with the ground.

2.3 Safety Considerations

Safety should always be a top priority when engaging in any form of exercise, including Wall Pilates. Here are some key safety considerations to keep in mind:

Consult Your Physician: Before starting any new exercise program, especially if you have underlying health conditions or concerns, consult with your healthcare provider to ensure that Wall Pilates is safe and appropriate for you.

Warm-Up: Always begin your Wall Pilates session with a gentle warm-up. This can include light stretching, deep breathing, and gentle movements to prepare your body for more intense exercises.

Proper Form: Pay close attention to your form and technique during Wall Pilates exercises. Proper alignment is crucial to prevent injury and maximize the benefits of each movement.

Listen to Your Body: Be mindful of your body's signals. If you experience pain or discomfort beyond the usual effort of the exercise, stop immediately and assess your form. Pushing through pain is not recommended.

Progress Gradually: If you're new to Wall Pilates, start with beginner-friendly exercises and progress at your own pace. Don't attempt advanced movements until you have built a solid foundation of strength and stability.

Stay Hydrated: Keep a water bottle nearby and stay hydrated throughout your practice to prevent dehydration.

Rest and Recovery: Incorporate rest days into your routine to allow your muscles to recover and prevent overtraining. Adequate rest is essential for long-term progress and injury prevention.

By setting up your practice space, having the necessary equipment, and adhering to safety considerations, you can embark on your Wall Pilates journey with confidence and peace of mind. These preparations will help create a conducive environment for your practice and minimize the risk of injuries or discomfort.

CHAPTER 3

Basic Principles of Pilates

3.1 Breathing

Breathing is one of the fundamental principles of Pilates and plays a central role in every movement. Proper breathing enhances the flow and efficiency of exercises while promoting relaxation and mindfulness. In Pilates, the emphasis is on lateral thoracic breathing, which means that you should inhale through your nose, expanding your ribcage outward and exhale through your mouth, drawing the ribs together. This type of breathing promotes better oxygenation of your muscles and helps engage your deep core muscles.

Breathing in Pilates serves several purposes:

- It aids in oxygenating the muscles, improving endurance and energy levels during exercises.

- It helps maintain stability and control during movements.

- Proper breathing promotes relaxation, reducing tension and stress.

- It enhances the mind-body connection, as you become more

aware of your breath and its relationship to your movements.

During Wall Pilates exercises, focus on coordinated breathing with your movements, maintaining a steady and controlled rhythm. Your breath should flow naturally and rhythmically to support the precision and control that Pilates exercises require.

3.2 Alignment

Alignment is another crucial principle of Pilates. It involves maintaining correct posture and body positioning throughout the exercises. Proper alignment ensures that your movements are effective, safe, and efficient. Wall Pilates, in particular, benefits from alignment principles, as the wall serves as a reference point for maintaining correct body positioning.

Key points of alignment in Wall Pilates include:

- Maintaining a neutral spine: Aligning the natural curves of the spine to avoid excessive arching or rounding during exercises.

- Proper head and neck positioning: Keeping the head aligned with the spine and avoiding undue strain on the neck.

- Engaging the core: Supporting the spine and promoting stability by engaging the core muscles.

- Aligning the limbs: Ensuring that the arms and legs are in the correct position relative to the body and the wall for each exercise.

Proper alignment in Wall Pilates minimizes the risk of injury, enhances the effectiveness of the exercises, and helps you build a strong foundation for more advanced movements.

3.3 Core Engagement

Core engagement is one of the core principles of Pilates and is integral to the effectiveness of Wall Pilates exercises. The core includes the muscles of the abdomen, lower back, and pelvis. Engaging the core is essential for maintaining stability, controlling movements, and protecting the spine. In Wall Pilates, the wall provides a unique opportunity to work on core strength with added support and feedback.

Key aspects of core engagement in Wall Pilates include:

- Activating the deep core muscles, such as the transversus abdominis and pelvic floor muscles.

- Creating a sense of length in the spine while keeping the core muscles engaged.

- Using the wall for support and feedback to maintain core stability during exercises.

Proper core engagement not only enhances the effectiveness of Wall Pilates exercises but also helps develop a strong and stable core that can benefit your overall posture and functional strength.

3.4 Concentration

Concentration, often referred to as mindfulness, is a fundamental principle in Pilates. It involves being fully present and mentally engaged in each movement. In Wall Pilates, concentration is particularly important because it helps you stay attuned to your body's alignment, sensations, and the quality of your movements.

The key aspects of concentration in Wall Pilates include:

- Focusing on the precise execution of each movement.

- Paying attention to your breath and its coordination with your exercises.

- Staying mentally engaged and avoiding distractions during your practice.

Concentration in Wall Pilates not only ensures the effectiveness of the exercises but also promotes a deeper mind-body connection, helping you maximize the benefits of your practice while reducing the risk of injury through focused, controlled movements.

3.5 Control

Control is another essential principle in Pilates, emphasizing the deliberate and precise execution of movements. In Wall Pilates, control is particularly important as it helps you maintain proper form and alignment while performing exercises. The concept of control extends to both the initiation and completion of each movement. Here's why control is crucial in Wall Pilates:

- Prevents jerky or uncontrolled movements that can lead to injury.

- Enhances the mind-body connection, as you actively engage your muscles to control each motion.

- Promotes the development of balanced and coordinated muscle strength.

Emphasizing control in Wall Pilates, you can ensure that your movements are purposeful, safe, and effective, ultimately leading to better results and a reduced risk of strain or injury.

3.6 Precision

Precision in Pilates is about performing each movement with exactness and attention to detail. It involves a focus on the specific muscles and alignment required for an exercise, avoiding unnecessary or extraneous movements. In Wall Pilates, the wall provides a valuable reference point for achieving precision in your movements:

- The wall can help you maintain consistent alignment and positioning throughout each exercise.

- By concentrating on precision, you target the intended muscle groups, making the exercises more effective.

- Precision leads to better control and balance, ultimately improving your overall performance and reducing the risk of injury.

Wall Pilates, with its support and guidance, allows you to refine your movements with precision, ensuring that you get the most out of each exercise while maintaining proper alignment and form.

3.7 Flow

Flow in Pilates refers to the seamless and fluid transition between movements and exercises. It encourages a sense of continuity and rhythm in your practice. In Wall Pilates, flow is essential for the following reasons:

- It promotes a graceful and connected quality to your movements, enhancing the overall experience.

- A continuous flow between exercises maintains your heart rate and body temperature, which can be important for cardiovascular fitness.

- Flow encourages you to stay present and engaged in your

practice, reducing the chance of distractions.

While precision and control are critical in Wall Pilates, flow ensures that your exercises are not mechanical or disjointed but rather a harmonious series of movements that work together to achieve your fitness and wellness goals. It also brings an element of grace and fluidity to your practice, making it enjoyable and satisfying.

CHAPTER 4

Wall Pilates Exercises

4.1 Warm-Up Exercises

Before you embark on the core Wall Pilates exercises, it's crucial to prepare your body and mind with a series of warm-up exercises. These warm-up exercises help increase blood flow, improve flexibility, and prepare your muscles for the more challenging movements that follow. Here are two essential warm-up exercises for Wall Pilates:

Standing Wall Roll Down

This exercise helps to mobilize your spine and gently stretch the hamstrings and back muscles.

Instructions:

1. Stand with your back against the wall, your heels about 4-6 inches away from the wall.

2. Your feet should be hip-width apart.

3. Begin by taking a deep breath in.

4. As you exhale, start to round your spine slowly, letting your head, neck, and upper back roll down toward the floor.

5. Keep your knees slightly bent to avoid overstretching your hamstrings.

6. Let your arms hang freely toward the floor.

7. Inhale at the bottom of the movement.

8. Exhale and slowly reverse the motion, rolling back up to a standing position, one vertebra at a time.

9. Repeat this movement several times to warm up your spine and improve flexibility.

Wall Hip Flexor Stretch

The Wall Hip Flexor Stretch is a fantastic way to release tension in the hip flexor muscles and prepare your body for core exercises.

Instructions:

1. Stand facing the wall with your feet hip-width apart.

2. Place your hands on the wall for support.

3. Take a step back with your right foot, about two to three feet away from the wall.

4. Keep your back leg straight and your toes pointing forward.

5. Bend your left knee and lean into the wall while keeping your back heel on the ground.

6. You should feel a stretch in the front of your right hip and thigh.

7. Hold the stretch for 20-30 seconds, breathing deeply.

8. Switch to the other leg and repeat the stretch.

These warm-up exercises prepare your body for the more challenging Wall Pilates exercises that follow. They also help to increase your range of motion and flexibility, making it easier to maintain proper form during the core strengthening exercises.

4.2 Core Strengthening Exercises

The core is a primary focus in Pilates, and Wall Pilates is no exception. These core strengthening exercises help you build a strong and stable core, which is essential for overall strength and balance.

Wall Plank

The Wall Plank is an excellent exercise for strengthening the core, shoulders, and arms.

Instructions:

1. Stand facing the wall, about an arm's length away.

2. Place your hands on the wall, shoulder-width apart, at chest height.

3. Step your feet back, keeping your body in a straight line from head to heels.

4. Engage your core and hold this position for 20-30 seconds or longer, if possible.

5. Be mindful of maintaining proper alignment with a neutral spine.

6. Gently lower yourself back to a standing position and repeat for multiple sets.

The Wall Plank provides a safe and effective way to develop core strength and improve your posture.

Wall Bridge

The Wall Bridge is designed to target the lower back, glutes, and core muscles.

Instructions:

1. Lie on your back with your feet against the wall, knees bent at a 90-degree angle.

2. Place your arms by your sides with your palms facing down.

3. Press your feet into the wall, lifting your hips off the floor.

4. Create a straight line from your shoulders to your knees.

5. Hold this position for 20-30 seconds while engaging your core and glutes.

6. Lower your hips back to the ground and repeat for multiple sets.

The Wall Bridge is a challenging exercise that helps strengthen the core and lower body while also improving hip stability.

These core strengthening exercises form the foundation of your Wall Pilates practice, and when performed regularly, they can lead to increased core strength, stability, and better overall posture. It's essential to maintain proper form and alignment during these exercises to maximize their effectiveness and reduce the risk of injury.

4.3 Upper Body Exercises

Upper body strength and mobility are important components of overall fitness, and Wall Pilates provides a unique platform for targeting these areas. Here are two upper body exercises that can be incorporated into your Wall Pilates routine:

Wall Push-Ups

Wall Push-Ups are a modified version of traditional push-ups that use the wall for support. This exercise is excellent for strengthening the chest, shoulders, and triceps.

Instructions:

1. Stand facing the wall at arm's length with your feet hip-width apart.

2. Place your hands on the wall at shoulder height and slightly wider than shoulder-width apart.

3. Step your feet back a little to create a slight incline.

4. Engage your core to maintain a straight line from head to heels.

5. Bend your elbows and lower your chest towards the wall.

6. Exhale as you push your body back to the starting position.

7. Complete 10-15 repetitions for one set, and aim for 2-3 sets.

Wall Push-Ups are an excellent way to build upper body strength and can be adapted to your fitness level by adjusting the distance from the wall. The closer you are to the wall, the easier the exercise; the farther away, the more challenging.

Wall Angels

Wall Angels are a fantastic exercise for improving shoulder mobility and posture.

Instructions:

1. Stand with your back against the wall, your feet hip-width apart, and your arms extended to the sides.

2. Press your back, arms, and hands flat against the wall.

3. Slowly slide your arms up the wall while keeping them in contact with the wall.

4. As you reach overhead, make sure your wrists, elbows, and shoulders stay in contact with the wall.

5. Return your arms to the starting position.

6. Repeat the movement for 10-15 repetitions for one set, aiming for 2-3 sets.

Wall Angels can help open up the chest, improve shoulder mobility, and counteract the effects of poor posture. They are a great addition to your Wall Pilates routine to enhance upper body flexibility and strength.

Including these upper body exercises in your Wall Pilates routine provides a comprehensive workout for your upper body, improving strength, mobility, and posture. As with all Pilates exercises, focus on proper form and alignment to reap the maximum benefits while minimizing the risk of injury.

4.4 Lower Body Exercises

Targeting the lower body is essential for developing strength, stability, and flexibility. Wall Pilates offers unique exercises to engage the muscles in your lower body effectively. Here are two lower body exercises for your Wall Pilates routine:

Wall Squats

Wall Squats are a fantastic exercise to strengthen the quadriceps, hamstrings, glutes, and calf muscles while improving lower body flexibility.

Instructions:

1. Stand with your back against the wall, your feet hip-width apart.

2. Place your hands on your hips or hold onto the wall for balance.

3. Slowly slide your back down the wall as you bend your knees, simulating a sitting position.

4. Continue lowering yourself until your thighs are parallel to the

ground, or as far as your flexibility allows.

5. Keep your knees aligned with your ankles and avoid letting them go beyond your toes.

6. Hold this position for a few seconds while engaging your leg muscles.

7. Slowly push yourself back up to a standing position.

8. Complete 10-15 repetitions for one set, aiming for 2-3 sets.

Wall Squats are an excellent way to develop lower body strength and stability while improving your squatting technique and form.

Wall Leg Lifts

Wall Leg Lifts are a great exercise for targeting the muscles in your lower abdomen, thighs, and hips.

Instructions:

1. Lie on your back with your buttocks against the wall, your legs extended, and your arms by your sides.

2. Press your lower back into the ground.

3. Lift your legs off the floor and extend them toward the ceiling, creating a 90-degree angle with your body.

4. Slowly lower your legs back down, keeping your lower back in contact with the floor.

5. Stop just before your feet touch the ground, then lift them back up.

6. Complete 10-15 repetitions for one set, aiming for 2-3 sets.

Wall Leg Lifts can help tone your lower abdominal muscles, strengthen your hip flexors, and enhance your lower body flexibility. They are an excellent exercise to add to your Wall Pilates routine for lower body strength and control.

Incorporating these lower body exercises into your Wall Pilates routine can provide a balanced and effective workout for your legs, glutes, and lower abdomen. Remember to maintain proper form and alignment to get the most out of these exercises while minimizing the risk of strain or injury.

4.5 Stretching and Cool Down

Stretching and cool-down exercises are essential components of any fitness routine, including Wall Pilates. They help improve flexibility, reduce muscle tension, and promote relaxation. Here are two stretching and cool-down exercises that can be included in your Wall Pilates routine:

Wall Chest Opener

The Wall Chest Opener is a wonderful stretch that helps counteract the effects of poor posture and relieve tension in the chest and shoulders.

Instructions:

1. Stand facing the wall, about an arm's length away.

2. Place your hands on the wall at shoulder height and slightly wider than shoulder-width apart.

3. Step one foot forward, creating a slight forward lean with your upper body.

4. Keep your body in a straight line
    from head to heel.

5. Gently lean into the wall,
    stretching your chest and front of
    the shoulders.

6. Hold the stretch for 20-30
    seconds, breathing deeply.

7. Switch your foot position and
    repeat the stretch to the other
    side.

The Wall Chest Opener is an excellent
way to release tension in the chest and
shoulders, and it can improve your
posture over time.

Wall Hamstring Stretch

The Wall Hamstring Stretch is a
fantastic way to improve the flexibility
of your hamstrings and relieve tension
in the lower back.

Instructions:

1. Lie on your back with your buttocks close to the wall.

2. Extend your legs upward, resting them against the wall.

3. Keep your legs straight but not locked, with your toes pointing toward the ceiling.

4. Let your arms rest by your sides.

5. Relax into this position, allowing gravity to gently stretch your hamstrings and lower back.

6. Hold the stretch for 20-30 seconds, breathing deeply and focusing on relaxing into the stretch.

The Wall Hamstring Stretch is a relaxing and effective way to improve the flexibility of your hamstrings and lower back, making it an ideal cool-down exercise.

Including these stretching and cool-
down exercises in your Wall Pilates
routine is essential for promoting
flexibility, reducing muscle tension,
and preventing post-exercise soreness.
These exercises also provide a calming
and restorative finish to your practice,
helping you unwind and relax after
your workout.

CHAPTER 5

Sample Wall Pilates Workouts

5.1. 15-Minute Beginner's Wall Pilates Routine

This 15-minute Wall Pilates routine is
designed for beginners and provides a
comprehensive introduction to Wall
Pilates exercises, focusing on core

strength, flexibility, and balance. Remember to maintain proper form and alignment throughout each exercise.

Warm-Up (2 minutes)

1. **Standing Wall Roll Down (1 minute)**

   - Stand with your back against the wall and feet hip-width apart.

   - Slowly roll down towards the floor while exhaling.

   - Inhale at the bottom, and exhale as you roll back up.

   - Repeat for 30 seconds.

2. **Wall Hip Flexor Stretch (1 minute)**

- Stand facing the wall, with one foot slightly behind the other.

- Bend your front knee and lean into the wall, feeling the stretch in your hip flexors.

- Hold for 30 seconds on each side.

Core Strengthening (4 minutes)

3. **Wall Plank (2 minutes)**

   - Stand facing the wall, place your hands at shoulder height, and step back.

   - Maintain a straight line from head to heels, engaging your core.

   - Hold for 1 minute.

4. **Wall Bridge (2 minutes)**

- Lie on your back with your feet against the wall and knees bent.

- Lift your hips off the floor, creating a straight line from your shoulders to your knees.

- Hold for 1 minute.

Upper Body (3 minutes)

5. **Wall Push-Ups (1.5 minutes)**

- Stand facing the wall, with your hands on the wall at shoulder height.

- Bend your elbows to perform push-ups while keeping your body in a straight line.

- Complete 10-12 repetitions.

6. **Wall Angels (1.5 minutes)**

   - Stand with your back against the wall, arms extended to the sides.

   - Slide your arms up the wall, maintaining contact with your hands, elbows, and shoulders.

   - Return to the starting position and repeat for 45 seconds.

Lower Body (3 minutes)

7. **Wall Squats (1.5 minutes)**

   - Stand facing the wall, slide down into a squat position while keeping your back against the wall.

- Return to the standing position, repeating for 45 seconds.

8. **Wall Leg Lifts (1.5 minutes)**

   - Lie on your back with your buttocks against the wall, and legs extended upward.

   - Lower your legs towards the wall while keeping your lower back on the floor.

   - Return to the starting position and repeat for 45 seconds.

Cool Down and Stretch (3 minutes)

9. **Wall Chest Opener (1.5 minutes)**

   - Stand facing the wall, place your hands on the

wall, and gently lean forward to stretch your chest and shoulders.

- Hold for 45 seconds on each side.

10. **Wall Hamstring Stretch (1.5 minutes)**

- Lie on your back with your legs extended upward against the wall, allowing gravity to stretch your hamstrings and lower back.

- Hold the stretch for 45 seconds.

This 15-minute beginner's Wall Pilates routine offers a well-rounded introduction to Wall Pilates exercises, targeting core strength, upper and lower body muscles, and promoting flexibility and balance. You can gradually increase the duration and complexity of exercises as you become more experienced with Wall Pilates.

5.2. 30-Minute Full-Body Wall Pilates Workout

This 30-minute Wall Pilates workout is designed to provide a comprehensive full-body workout for intermediate to advanced practitioners. It combines core strength, upper and lower body exercises, and stretching for a balanced routine. Ensure proper form and alignment during each exercise.

Warm-Up (4 minutes)

1. **Standing Wall Roll Down (2 minutes)**

   - Stand with your back against the wall and feet hip-width apart.

   - Slowly roll down toward the floor while exhaling.

- Inhale at the bottom and exhale as you roll back up.

- Repeat for 1 minute.

2. **Wall Hip Flexor Stretch (2 minutes)**

   - Stand facing the wall with one foot slightly behind the other.

   - Bend your front knee and lean into the wall, feeling the stretch in your hip flexors.

   - Hold for 1 minute on each side.

Core Strengthening (8 minutes)

3. **Wall Plank (4 minutes)**

   - Stand facing the wall, place your hands at

shoulder height, and step back.

- Maintain a straight line from head to heels, engaging your core.

- Hold for 2 minutes.

4. **Wall Bridge (4 minutes)**

- Lie on your back with your feet against the wall and knees bent.

- Lift your hips off the floor, creating a straight line from your shoulders to your knees.

- Hold for 2 minutes.

Upper Body (6 minutes)

5. **Wall Push-Ups (3 minutes)**

- Stand facing the wall, with your hands on the wall at shoulder height.

- Bend your elbows to perform push-ups while keeping your body in a straight line.

- Complete 15-20 repetitions.

6. **Wall Angels (3 minutes)**

- Stand with your back against the wall, arms extended to the sides.

- Slide your arms up the wall, maintaining contact with your hands, elbows, and shoulders.

- Return to the starting position and repeat for 1.5 minutes.

7. **Wall Squats (4 minutes)**

- Stand facing the wall, slide down into a squat position while keeping your back against the wall.

- Return to the standing position, repeating for 2 minutes.

8. **Wall Leg Lifts (4 minutes)**

- Lie on your back with your buttocks against the wall and legs extended upward.

- Lower your legs toward the wall while keeping your lower back on the floor.

- Return to the starting position and repeat for 2 minutes.

Cool Down and Stretch (4 minutes)

9. **Wall Chest Opener (2 minutes)**

   - Stand facing the wall, place your hands on the wall, and gently lean forward to stretch your chest and shoulders.

   - Hold for 1 minute on each side.

10. **Wall Hamstring Stretch (2 minutes)**

    - Lie on your back with your legs extended upward against the wall, allowing gravity to stretch your hamstrings and lower back.

- Hold the stretch for 1 minute.

This 30-minute full-body Wall Pilates workout is ideal for intermediate to advanced practitioners seeking a comprehensive and challenging routine. It targets core strength, upper and lower body muscles, and flexibility while providing a well-rounded workout. Adjust the intensity and duration of exercises as needed to suit your fitness level and goals.

CHAPTER 6

Progression and Challenges

6.1 Advancing Your Wall Pilates Practice

Progressing in your Wall Pilates practice is an exciting journey that can lead to increased strength, flexibility, and overall well-being. Here are some tips for advancing your practice and taking on new challenges:

1. Gradual Progression:

- Start with the basics and gradually add complexity to your routine. As you become more comfortable with the exercises, increase the number of repetitions or hold positions for longer.

2. Incorporate Variations:

- Explore variations of Wall Pilates exercises to challenge different muscle groups. For example, modify the Wall Plank by lifting one leg, or intensify Wall Push-Ups by using an incline bench for a steeper angle.

3. Resistance and Props:

- Consider adding resistance bands or small weights to certain exercises for increased intensity. This can help you build more strength and muscle endurance.

4. Balance and Stability:

- Integrate balance and stability challenges into your practice by performing exercises on one leg or with your eyes closed. This can enhance your proprioception and core strength.

5. Deepen Mind-Body Connection:

- Focus on refining your breathing and concentration. Pay attention to the sensations in your body during each exercise, and connect with your breath to enhance your mind-body connection.

6. Personalized Routine:

- Tailor your Wall Pilates routine to address your specific fitness goals and needs. Whether you're aiming for increased flexibility, core strength, or pain relief, customize your practice accordingly.

7. Professional Guidance:

- Consider working with a certified Pilates instructor. They can provide personalized guidance, correct your form, and create a structured plan for your progression.

8. Consistency is Key:

- Regular practice is essential for progress. Aim for a consistent schedule, even if it means shorter sessions. A little practice often can yield better results than infrequent, long sessions.

9. Record Your Progress:

- Keep a journal to track your progress. Note your achievements, improvements, and areas that still need work. This can help you stay motivated and see how far you've come.

10. Listen to Your Body:

- Pay attention to your body's signals. If you experience pain or discomfort, it's essential to stop and assess your form. Don't push yourself too hard and risk injury.

11. Stay Open to Learning:

- Wall Pilates, like all forms of Pilates, is a practice that continuously evolves. Stay open to learning new techniques and approaches to enhance your practice.

Advancing your Wall Pilates practice is a gradual and rewarding process. With dedication and commitment, you can enjoy the physical and mental benefits of Wall Pilates while challenging yourself to reach new levels of strength, flexibility, and overall well-being.

6.2 Common Mistakes in Wall Pilates and How to Avoid Them

Wall Pilates is a fantastic exercise method, but like any form of fitness, there are common mistakes that people make. Being aware of these mistakes and knowing how to avoid them can help you get the most out of your Wall Pilates practice while reducing the risk of injury. Here are some common mistakes and how to avoid them:

1. Poor Alignment and Posture:

- **Mistake:** Allowing your body to sag or slouch during exercises or not aligning your spine properly against the wall.

- **Avoidance:** Prioritize maintaining proper alignment and posture. Use the wall as a reference point to ensure your body is in the correct position. Engage your core to support your spine and avoid sagging.

2. Overarching the Lower Back:

- **Mistake:** Arching your lower back excessively during exercises, especially when doing Wall Bridges.

- **Avoidance:** Focus on maintaining a neutral spine. Engage your core muscles and keep your lower back in contact with the wall or floor. Avoid hyperextension to prevent straining your lower back.

3. Neglecting Breathing:

- **Mistake:** Holding your breath or not coordinating your breath with your movements.

- **Avoidance:** Pay close attention to your breath. Inhale through your nose to expand your ribcage and exhale through your mouth to engage your core muscles. A consistent and controlled breathing pattern is crucial for proper execution.

4. Using Too Much Momentum:

- **Mistake:** Relying on momentum to complete exercises rather than engaging your muscles.

- **Avoidance:** Perform movements with control and precision. Focus on the muscles you're targeting, and avoid jerky or fast-paced movements. Quality and control should always come before quantity.

5. Skipping the Warm-Up and Cool Down:

- **Mistake:** Neglecting to warm up and cool down properly.

- **Avoidance:** Always start your Wall Pilates session with a warm-up to prepare your body and finish with a cool-down to stretch and relax your muscles. These phases are crucial for injury prevention and recovery.

6. Pushing Through Pain:

- **Mistake:** Ignoring pain or discomfort and pushing through exercises that your body is not ready for.

- **Avoidance:** Listen to your body. If an exercise causes pain or discomfort beyond the usual effort, stop immediately and assess your form. It's essential to progress gradually and avoid overexertion.

7. Inadequate Safety Considerations:

- **Mistake:** Neglecting safety considerations, such as consulting a healthcare provider if you have underlying health issues.

- **Avoidance:** Prioritize safety by consulting a healthcare provider before starting Wall Pilates, especially if you have any medical conditions or concerns. Always follow safety guidelines and recommendations.

8. Lack of Variation:

- **Mistake:** Sticking to the same routine without introducing variety.

- **Avoidance:** Include a variety of exercises and progressions in your Wall Pilates routine to challenge different muscle groups and prevent plateaus. This will keep your practice engaging and effective.

By avoiding these common mistakes and staying mindful of your form and body's signals, you can enjoy the full benefits of Wall Pilates while minimizing the risk of injury or ineffective workouts.

6.3 Can Wall Pilates Help with Posture?

Yes, Wall Pilates can be highly effective in improving and maintaining good posture. Posture is influenced by the strength and flexibility of various muscle groups, especially those in the core, back, and neck. Wall Pilates targets these muscle groups and focuses on enhancing overall body awareness, making it a valuable tool for posture improvement. Here's how Wall Pilates can help with posture:

1. **Core Strength:** Wall Pilates places a significant emphasis on core strength, particularly the deep core muscles like the transversus abdominis. A strong core helps support your spine and prevents excessive arching or rounding, which can lead to poor posture.

2. **Alignment Awareness:** Wall Pilates encourages proper alignment of the spine and limbs. Practicing exercises with your back against the wall helps you become more aware of your body's positioning and how it should feel in an aligned posture.

3. **Spine Mobility:** Wall Pilates exercises often involve spinal movements that promote flexibility and mobility in the spine. Improved spine mobility can help reduce stiffness and discomfort associated with poor posture.

4. **Strengthening Postural Muscles:** Wall Pilates targets the muscles responsible for maintaining good posture, such as the muscles in the upper back, shoulders, and neck. Strengthening these muscles can

help you stand and sit more upright.

5. **Breathing and Relaxation:** Proper breathing techniques are essential in Wall Pilates. Learning to coordinate your breath with movements can help you relax tense muscles and improve your overall body awareness, including posture.

6. **Body Awareness:** Wall Pilates encourages mindfulness and body awareness. By focusing on your form and how your body feels during exercises, you develop a better understanding of your posture and can actively make adjustments to maintain good posture.

7. **Post-Workout Stretching:** Wall Pilates typically includes stretching and cool-down

exercises that target areas
commonly affected by poor
posture, such as the chest,
shoulders, and hamstrings.

To get the most benefit for your
posture, it's important to maintain a
regular Wall Pilates practice.
Consistency is key to making lasting
improvements. As with any exercise
program, it's also a good idea to consult
with a certified Pilates instructor or a
physical therapist to receive
personalized guidance and exercises
tailored to your specific posture-related
needs and any existing postural issues
or imbalances. Additionally, you can
apply the principles learned in Wall
Pilates to your everyday activities and
work on maintaining proper posture
throughout the day.

6.4 How Often Should I Do Wall Pilates?

The frequency at which you should practice Wall Pilates depends on your fitness goals, your current fitness level, and the time you can dedicate to your workouts. Here are some general guidelines to help you determine how often to do Wall Pilates:

1. **Beginners:** If you're new to Wall Pilates or exercise in general, it's a good idea to start with 2-3 sessions per week. This frequency allows your body to adapt to the exercises and minimizes the risk of overuse injuries.

2. **Intermediate to Advanced Practitioners:** For those with some experience in Wall Pilates or a similar exercise regimen, 3-5 sessions per week can be

suitable. This frequency provides opportunities for skill improvement and strength development.

3. **Maintenance:** If you're using Wall Pilates primarily for maintenance and posture improvement, 2-4 sessions per week should suffice. Consistency is key to maintaining the benefits of your practice.

4. **Rehabilitation or Specific Goals:** If you're using Wall Pilates as part of a rehabilitation program or to achieve specific fitness goals, your frequency may vary. In such cases, it's crucial to consult with a healthcare provider or a certified Pilates instructor who can provide personalized guidance.

5. **Balanced Schedule:** Consider mixing Wall Pilates with other forms of exercise to maintain a balanced fitness routine. Combining Pilates with cardio, strength training, and flexibility exercises can provide comprehensive benefits.

Remember that the quality of your practice is more important than quantity. Ensure that you perform Wall Pilates exercises with proper form and alignment, and prioritize consistency. Over time, you can adjust your frequency based on how your body responds and your evolving fitness goals.

6.5 Is Wall Pilates Suitable for Everyone?

Wall Pilates is generally suitable for a wide range of individuals, but there are some considerations to keep in mind:

1. **Beginners:** Wall Pilates can be adapted for beginners, with the use of simpler exercises and modifications. It's a great way to introduce individuals to the world of Pilates.

2. **Intermediate to Advanced Practitioners:** Wall Pilates can be adjusted to challenge more experienced practitioners. It offers a variety of exercises and progressions to keep workouts engaging and challenging.

3. **Rehabilitation:** Wall Pilates can be used in rehabilitation programs to improve strength

and flexibility. However, individuals with specific injuries or medical conditions should consult with a healthcare provider or a certified Pilates instructor to ensure that exercises are appropriate and safe.

4. **Pregnancy:** Wall Pilates can be adapted for pregnant individuals, but it's important to work with a qualified instructor who is experienced in prenatal Pilates. Some exercises may need to be modified or avoided during pregnancy.

5. **Medical Conditions:** Individuals with certain medical conditions, such as severe osteoporosis or cardiovascular issues, should seek medical clearance and guidance from a healthcare provider or physical

therapist before starting Wall
Pilates.

6. **Individual Goals:** Wall Pilates
   can be tailored to different
   fitness goals, including
   improving posture, core strength,
   flexibility, and overall well-
   being.

While Wall Pilates is generally
accessible to many, it's essential to
approach it with mindfulness and
safety. Consult with a certified Pilates
instructor if you're new to Pilates or
have specific concerns. They can create
a personalized program that considers
your individual needs and goals.
Additionally, they can ensure that you
perform exercises correctly, reducing
the risk of injury and maximizing the
benefits of your practice.

www.ingramcontent.com/pod-product-compliance
Lightning Source LLC
Chambersburg PA
CBHW050841260726
48660CB00006B/2363